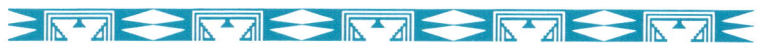

TABLE OF CONTENTS

INTRODUCTION 3

ALERT PROGRAM GOALS 5

BASICS OF THE ALERT PROGRAM 5

    OCCUPATIONAL THERAPY 5

    SENSORY INTEGRATION 6

    AROUSAL STATES OR ENGINE LEVELS 8

    PROTECTIVE RESPONSES
    OF THE NERVOUS SYSTEM 11

    INHIBITION AND ITS RELATIONSHIP
    TO "HEAVY WORK" 12

    SENSORY-MOTOR PREFERENCES 14

    "DETECTIVE WORK" 16

STAGES OF TEACHING THE ALERT PROGRAM 17

REFERENCES 22

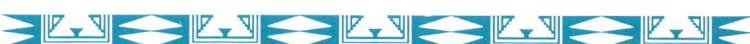

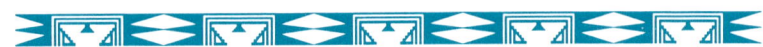

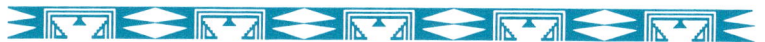

INTRODUCTION

It has been our experience that children have an innate ability to guide us to empower them, if only we listen. By way of example, the core of the Alert Program was taught to Mary Sue by one of her instructors, an 11 year old client. This child entered each therapy session appearing to be lethargic, disinterested, and resistant to activities or interactions (in a low arousal state). After a short period of active play, she became alert, communicative, confident, energetic, and enthusiastic (in an optimal arousal state). Despite this dramatic change during therapy, the child would return for her next therapy session in the same low arousal state and reportedly there was little carry-over to home or school.

It became apparent to Mary Sue that the child needed to understand her own arousal states in order to generalize the effects of therapy. Mary Sue began to explain this to her client by saying, "If your body is like a car engine, sometimes it runs on low, sometimes it runs on high, and sometimes it runs just right."

In subsequent therapy sessions, Mary Sue and her client played together and shared their inner experiences of arousal states through the framework of the engine vocabulary. Mary Sue listened carefully to the guidance that the child offered in learning about self-regulation. The 11 year old blossomed into a child who learned how to take responsibility for herself and made great gains in building self-confidence and self-esteem. Through interactions with this child and the many children who followed, the Alert Program was developed.

The program promotes awareness of how individuals regulate their arousal states and encourages the use of sensory-motor strategies. Consisting of a series of lessons and activities, the program helps children learn to monitor and change their levels of alertness appropriate to a situation or task. Though initially designed for children 8 to 12, the program has been adapted for preschool through high school students, and for adults. In addition, it has been implemented in a variety of settings including classroom, home, camp and private practice.

We believe all behavior has meaning and that it is our responsibility to seek out what children might be communicating to us through their behavior. The leader's job is to introduce the concepts and facilitate the program while vigilantly watching for children's self-initiated modifications. Children will adjust the vocabulary and offer activities to make the program work for them.

We strongly encourage parents and teachers to participate in the program. The primary adults in the students' lives need to have an understanding of the program's theory, engine vocabulary, and strategies. Supportive adults who understand the Alert Program concepts are fundamental to students' success.

We have had years of positive experiences using the Alert Program and watching students learn about self-regulation through play and discussions. One of our greatest joys is to work with children as they discover their own answers to the question, "How does your engine run?"

Mary Sue Williams   Sherry Shellenberger

ACKNOWLEDGEMENTS

We gratefully acknowledge Patti Oetter's influence and guidance, for without her help, the Alert Program would not have been conceived. We would like to express our deep appreciation to the staff who worked at Albuquerque Therapy Services in 1987 through 1989 (Lynn Anaya Atkins, Donna Cizmadia, Mary Hartley, Marci Laurel, Carla Cay Neimeyer, Hillary Phelps, Kathy Taylor, Maryann Trott, and Sue Windeck.) They helped to expand the concepts and added greatly to the details of the program. An additional and special thanks to Steve Cool, Marci Laurel, Eileen Richter, Helen Rynaski, and Maryann Trott for their support, suggestions and assistance in editing. Finally, we recognize and cherish the children with whom we have worked, for they have been our finest teachers.

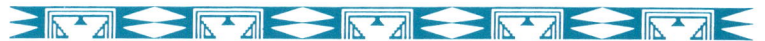

ALERT PROGRAM GOALS

The Alert Program is designed to:

- teach children, parents, and teachers how to recognize arousal states as they relate to attention, learning, and behavior.

- help children recognize and expand the number of self-regulation strategies they use in a variety of tasks and settings.

- give therapists, parents, and teachers a framework (vocabulary, activities, and environments) to help children recognize and regulate their own arousal states.

- help parents and teachers understand that behavior may reflect the student's best attempt to respond adaptively and efficiently to the demands of a situation or task.

BASICS OF THE ALERT PROGRAM

The Alert Program is most useful when those involved have a working knowledge of the underlying concepts. The eight key concepts used in the program are identified and defined in the following pages.

OCCUPATIONAL THERAPY

"Occupational therapy is a health profession concerned with improving a person's occupational performance. In a pediatric setting, the occupational therapist deals with children whose occupations are usually players, preschoolers, or students" (*A Parent's Guide to Understanding Sensory Integration*, 1986).

Occupational therapists use a knowledge base of neurology, anatomy, physiology, kinesiology, child development, psychology, psychosocial development, activity-task analysis, and therapeutic techniques. They are

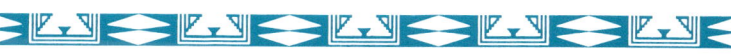

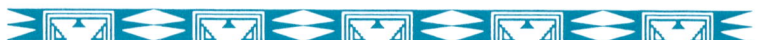

trained to treat clients holistically, addressing their cognitive, emotional, and physical needs through functional, activity-based treatment. When working in pediatrics, occupational therapists select activities that are of interest and have meaning for children, and that also meet therapeutic goals.

SENSORY INTEGRATION

For over 30 years, Dr. A. Jean Ayres brought together her knowledge of neuroscience and occupational therapy to pioneer and create the theory, assessments, and treatment principles of sensory integration. Sensory Integration International teaches that, "Play is the work of children. Through play, children learn about themselves and the world around them. When all they see, hear, and feel make sense to them, the process of sensory integration occurs." Children have an innate drive to move, explore, and learn through pleasurable experiences. Therapy sessions that children perceive as fun, motivating, and playful are essential to the therapeutic process.

An analogy of a computer can be used to describe sensory integration [Fig. 1]. To write a letter, information is typed into a computer (input). The computer processes the information and a hard copy of the work (printed piece of paper) can be produced (output). When an error is detected in the letter, one possibility is that the information was typed incorrectly (input). If no error is found there, one might conclude that the cause of the error was in the internal processing of the computer.

Similarly, a parent or teacher may observe problems in a child's attention, motor coordination, impulse control, activity level, or ability to experience, learn, and interact with the environment or others (output). An occupational therapist may be asked to evaluate the child for sensory integration difficulties. The occupational therapist first considers perception and registration of sensory-motor information; what the child sees, hears, touches, tastes, and smells, in addition to how movement and gravity are experienced (input). To determine how the child's brain is processing this input, the therapist gathers information through clinical observations, sensory history, and standardized tests.

The therapist asks how the child responds to a variety of sensory-motor experiences. Can the child use sensory-motor experiences to learn, interact,

Figure 1

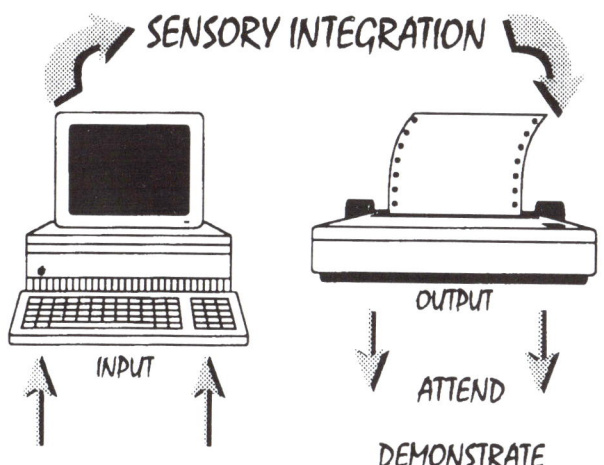

SENSORY INTEGRATION

INPUT

OUTPUT
ATTEND

WHAT WE:
SEE
HEAR
TOUCH
TASTE
SMELL

DEMONSTRATE KNOWLEDGE

LEARN

INTERACT WITH OTHERS

INTERTACT WITH THE ENVIRONMENT

MOVE

HOW WE EXPERIENCE:
MOVEMENT
GRAVITY

HAVE SELF-ESTEEM

HAVE SELF-CONTROL

EXPRESS FEELINGS

FEEDBACK

© 1992 TherapyWorks, Inc.

explore, and demonstrate knowledge? Does the child respond negatively or with extreme behaviors (flight, fright, or fight responses) to unexpected or light touch, unstable surfaces, loud noises, visual distractions, or certain tastes, textures, and smells? Can the child filter out irrelevant sensory input? For example, can the child attend to the sound of a teacher's voice rather than the heater fan?

AROUSAL STATES OR ENGINE LEVELS

"Arousal" can be considered a state of the nervous system, describing how alert one feels. To attend, concentrate, and perform tasks in a manner suitable to the situational demands, one's nervous system must be in an optimal state of arousal for that particular task (Mercer & Snell, 1977). The word "alert" is used rather than "arousal" when explaining this program to students. It quickly will become apparent (especially working with preadolescents) that the word "alert" should be used to avoid any distractions that could easily be created by the word "arousal"! Through the years, this choice of words has proven to be a wise one.

The first chart in figure 2 is an example of a normal adult nervous system. Upon rising, Anne finds it difficult to get up and get going. Anne is not in need of more sleep, but her engine is running in low gear. She takes a shower and eats. By the time she gets to work, Anne's nervous system is in an optimal state of alertness (just right for work). This allows for concentration and the efficient accomplishment of work tasks. At about 10:00 a.m., Anne is anticipating a coffee break because she has been sitting in a business meeting and is plummeting into low gear. During the day Anne experiences a drop in productivity after lunch and again at about 3:00 p.m. She arrives home at 5:30 p.m. Her children are arguing, and she is rushing to get dinner in order to make a 6:15 p.m. meeting. Her engine is rising toward high gear. She makes it to her meeting and welcomes the opportunity to go to bed at 10:00 p.m., to drop into a state of sleep.

The second example is that of a child whose engine is typically in high alert. Paul usually pops out of bed and immediately is in motion. His state fluctuates slightly, but he remains in high gear throughout the day. Paul has poor attention in class and frequently has difficulty getting along with others.

Figure 2

EXAMPLES OF ENGINE LEVELS

Normal Day (Anne)

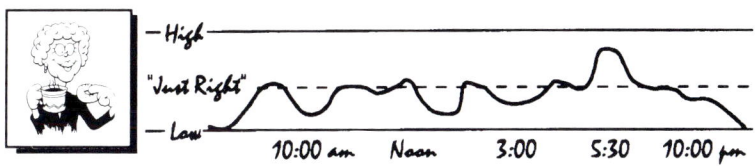

High (Paul)

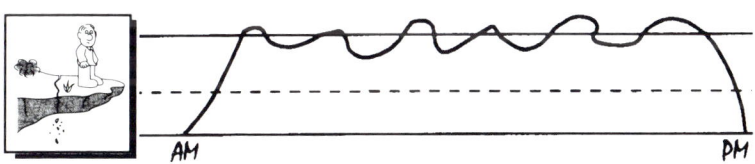

Low (Carl)

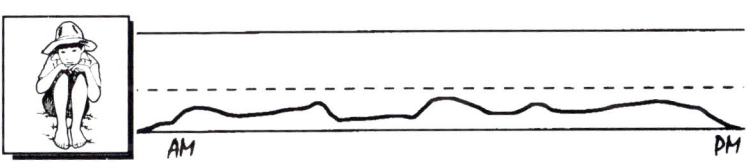

He has been described as "hyper," "antsy," and having a "motor mouth." At bedtime, it is very hard for Paul to fall asleep. It is difficult to transition from his engine running at a high speed to the lowest state of sleep.

A child whose engine usually runs in the low range is illustrated in the third example. Carl slowly rises out of bed after several reminders and, eventually, threats from his parents. He seems to remain lethargic throughout the day, finding it very difficult to complete his assignments at school. Carl can become restless and fidgety after long periods of seat work. His teacher does not consider him to be a behavior problem but notes that she has problems motivating Carl. He is described by his mother as quiet and occasionally irritable. Carl can fall asleep quite easily.

"Self-regulation" is the ability to attain, maintain, and change arousal appropriately for a task or situation. Paul and Carl are having difficulties with self-regulation. Often, they are unable to change the degree of alertness they feel; therefore, they have trouble functioning optimally.

In the Alert Program, children learn to identify their own arousal states. In an effort to keep this program simple for students, only what their engine feels like or observed behavior is labeled. A child's engine may appear to be running at a high speed, when actually the nervous system is in a state of low arousal and the child is demonstrating "hyperactive" behaviors in an attempt to self-regulate (Zentall & Zentall, 1983).

For example, a young boy stays up past his bedtime because a special friend is visiting. The child may be falling into a low state of arousal, but in an effort to not miss out, he may run around the room, jump, or talk excessively. It would be helpful to tell the boy that his engine is running on high and offer other ways to obtain an optimal level of functioning so that he can enjoy his time with his friend. To explain to the child that his actual arousal state may be in low would most likely confuse him. The adult, however, should note that behavior appearing to be hyperactive may actually be an attempt by the child's nervous system to avoid going into a lower state of arousal. It is important to keep this in mind when suggesting appropriate sensory-motor strategies to regulate arousal states.

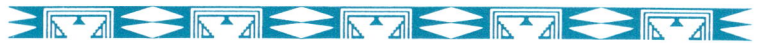

PROTECTIVE RESPONSES OF THE NERVOUS SYSTEM

When adults are concerned about a student's behavior, one possible cause to consider is the nervous system's response to sensory information. Behaviors that seem out of proportion to a situation (such as hitting, crying, or running away) actually may be protective responses of the brain. Protective responses are <u>automatic</u>, and are elicited without cognitive thought. The protective responses that will be discussed in detail are sensory defensiveness and flight, fright, or fight reactions.

"Sensory defensiveness is simply the over activation of our protective senses" (Wilbarger & Wilbarger, 1991). These individuals' nervous systems may be overly sensitive to loud noises, excessive amounts of visual input, unexpected touch, certain types of movement, unsteady surfaces, and certain types of food textures, tastes, and smells.

Consider how a person lost at night in an unfamiliar city might react to hearing sudden footsteps and feeling a touch on the hand. The brain would receive messages from the auditory and tactile systems and make connections to several other parts of the brain. A message would then be sent to the autonomic nervous system preparing the body to protect itself. For example, the person may begin to breathe quick shallow breaths. The blood supply would decrease to the limbs and increase to the heart. The heart would start beating faster. Blood pressure and body temperature would rise. The body would react in an automatic way with either a flight, fright, or fight reaction. The person responding in a flight reaction might run away. A fright reaction might cause the person to freeze and not move. In a fight reaction, the person might lash out and hit or kick. All these responses are appropriate when personal danger is perceived.

If a child is standing in line at school and is touched from behind, however, it is not appropriate to react by hitting, running away, or crying hysterically. What happens at this point? The teacher approaches and says, "You know the rules! Why did you hit another student?" The child is not able to say, "I do know the rules, but my brain perceived personal danger in response to this sensory input and decided, in error, to send messages to my autonomic nervous system to prepare my body to go into flight, fright or fight for protection."

A flight, fright, or fight reaction can occur in more subtle ways. In a

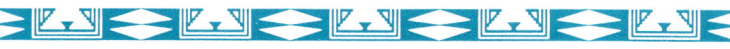

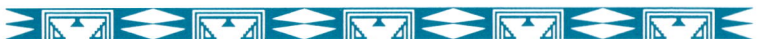

fight response, one might not physically hit but rather verbally fight by refusing to participate in an activity, by being irritable or by saying, "No!" Instead of running away, a subtle flight response may be seen in a child turning away from an activity that the body interprets as dangerous. In a fright response, a child may say "I can't," cry, or express fear in a way that seems to be out of proportion to the situation. It is, however, in proportion to how the child perceives the sensory input.

Obviously, not every child who hits, runs away, or cries is experiencing sensory defensiveness or a flight, fright, or fight reaction, but any nervous system will respond to protect the body if the brain's *perception* is that of danger. To an observer, this reaction may seem extreme, but the brain's first priority is protection of the body. Therefore, a real threat or perceived threat (based on present or past experience) is handled in the same way. A perceived threat is *real* to the perceiver, and it needs to be honored as his or her truth.

INHIBITION AND ITS RELATIONSHIP TO "HEAVY WORK"

*I*n order to understand the sensory-motor strategies that will be suggested to help students self-regulate, the concepts of inhibition and the effects of "heavy work" (or proprioceptive input from muscles and joints) must be understood.

Consider the brain. The top part of the brain is called the cortex and is responsible for our thinking. The center section is called the brain stem and contains the reticular formation. It is a very old section of the brain and is responsible, in part, for how alert one feels. The back section of the brain is called the cerebellum. One of its jobs is to take in information, called proprioceptive input, from muscles and joints. The brain parts are not important, but knowing how they work together will help in understanding the role of proprioceptive input in the Alert Program.

For example, Mary's engine is in high gear when she comes in from recess at school. If her teacher states that everyone has to get their seat work completed in order to go on the field trip tomorrow, Mary may use the top part of her brain to try to get her engine in an optimal state to do her work. She might try to talk to herself to stay on task and remind herself of the consequence if she does not complete her work. From the top of her brain

(cortex) down, she is trying to inhibit herself or use "top-down inhibition." This is not an efficient way to concentrate or self-regulate and is most likely not possible for an entire school day.

A more efficient way is to engage the back part of the brain. If one can engage this part of the brain, it will send messages to the center part of the brain, which in turn, will help the body attain an optimal arousal state or engine level. One of the ways that the back part of the brain can be engaged is through heavy work of the body's muscles and joints. This is called "bottom-up inhibition", because the brain receives input from the body.

If a teacher notices that Mary's engine is running in high, she might suggest that Mary carry a heavy box to the office before beginning her seat work. The teacher would be helping to send messages from the back part of the brain to the center part. Through "bottom-up inhibition" with heavy work to her muscles and joints, Mary would most likely return with her engine running just right. She would be in an optimal arousal state to complete her seat work.

In summary, the Alert Program teaches ways to utilize the more efficient bottom-up inhibition through sensory-motor strategies, rather than relying on top-down inhibition which uses ineffective verbal reminders such as asking the student to "get in control." If one can set up the nervous system with a "sensory diet" (Wilbarger and Wilbarger, 1991) of proprioceptive input, along with other sensory-motor input (vision, hearing, motion, and touch), the student's nervous system has the best chance of functioning optimally.

The back part of the brain is stimulated through heavy work to muscles and joints. There are many ways for the brain to receive this type of proprioceptive input: pushing and pulling games, lifting or carrying heavy objects, wrestling, playing football, moving furniture, biking, hoeing in the garden, taking out the trash, and "tug-of-war." More subtle ways are pushing hands together, standing and pushing against a desk with hands and arms, stretching, doing a "chair push-up" (lifting one's body off the chair seat, with hands grasping the sides of the seat, and straightening the elbows), manipulating stiff putty, and lying under heavy quilts or pillows. Also, one can feel heavy work in the jaw joint and muscles around the jaw by chewing gum (some need to chew several pieces at one time), chewing on erasers, eating crunchy foods, or pulling and chewing on a straw. All these types of proprioceptive input are very useful in helping the brain to regulate arousal

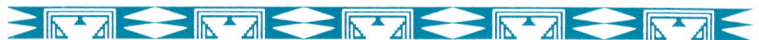

states.

The same proprioceptive input can have both calming and alerting effects, so it can be used when engines are either too high or too low. Unlike other sensory inputs, proprioceptive input is rarely overloading to a nervous system. It is, therefore, an excellent strategy to use to excite or inhibit engine levels. Teachers and parents, with knowledge of arousal states, can offer these types of activities to children. For example, a teacher may observe that before a spelling test, some of her students' engines are running in low speed and others in high speed. The teacher could suggest that the whole class stand up and push on their desks with their hands, or stretch.

Although it may sound complex, top-down and bottom-up inhibition are frequently utilized and necessary, in daily life. It is perhaps a common experience to be in a situation where young children are excited. On a recent trip to the Ice Capades, one such child was told, "If you don't stay in your seat, we'll have to leave!" The child then proceeded to kick the back of the chair, immediately in front. The occupant of the seat being kicked would probably take small comfort in knowing that the child was using proprioceptive input and bottom-up inhibition to self-regulate. The occupant could employ top-down inhibition to remember that it would only be a short time before the child would choose another sensory-motor strategy such as chewing a piece of gum.

SENSORY-MOTOR PREFERENCES

Attaining, maintaining, and/or changing arousal states is often an unconscious process. Teachers, therapists, and parents need to develop skills in observing, understanding, and respecting their own and their students' sensory-motor preferences, in order to direct learning. (Patricia Oetter, Patricia Wilbarger, and Julia Wilbarger are gratefully recognized as the originators of valuable information regarding the role of sensory-motor input in self-regulation.)

Determining sensory-motor preferences helps to assess what strategies may be most useful in achieving and maintaining an appropriate arousal state for various tasks and situations. What supports or compromises a person's performance? Observe how much, how often, and for how long a person engages in sensory-motor experiences. Everyone has an innate drive to seek

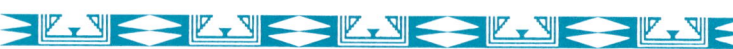

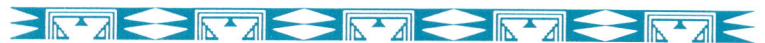

and receive the sensory-motor input their bodies and brains need. As the normal nervous system matures, this inner drive remains, but the degree of intensity, duration, and frequency of sensory-motor experiences changes and usually decreases (Cool & Oetter, 1990).

For example, a child's nervous system may "crave" swinging. In a certain developmental period, a child may choose to swing at every school recess (frequency), pumping as hard and as fast as possible (intensity). The child may continue swinging the whole recess period (duration). The adult's nervous system may enjoy swinging but only seeks slight swinging movements (intensity) for short periods of time (duration), once in a great while (frequency). Most adult nervous systems do not need as much intensity, frequency, or duration of sensory-motor input to reach or maintain optimal functioning (arousal) appropriate for a specific task or situation.

This principle can be understood by comparing the amount of sensory-motor input needed by an adult and a child to maintain attention while listening to a lecture. An individual who is interested in the lecture will use oral motor input, movement, or touch experiences to maintain alertness. At any age, the nervous system needs a sensory diet in order to maintain attention (Wilbarger & Wilbarger, 1991). Some common strategies that an adult might use include fidgeting with jewelry, sucking on the lip or the inside of the mouth, putting fingers near the mouth or chin, shifting in the chair, or slightly swinging or bouncing one leg (while seated with legs crossed at the knee). In a similar situation, a child may need far greater input to sustain attention. The child may chew and/or twist hair, suck on fingers or on a collar, tip the chair back on two legs to rock, and frequently change positions ("wiggle" or "squirm") to maintain arousal.

Unfortunately, some adults believe that if children are moving about they cannot be paying attention. The old command, "Sit still and pay attention," is still heard in many homes and classrooms. To the contrary, most children can *either* sit still *or* pay attention. They *need* to move to get sensory-motor input *in order* to pay attention.

The adult's slight movements while listening are rarely considered a sign of inattention because they are socially accepted and less obvious. Adult sensory-motor experiences used to achieve and maintain an appropriate level of alertness to attend are often referred to as idiosyncrasies or habits. An adult's loved ones are most aware of which sensory-motor habits are being

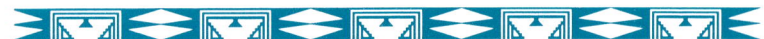

utilized. This can often be a topic for discussion (or argument), such as this case described by a teacher.

"I jingle and play with coins in my pocket, when I am listening to my wife describe her day. My wife gets irritated and tells me to stop. Who's right?" No one is right or wrong! Understanding that sensory-motor experiences have a purpose often leads to increased acceptance and understanding of others' actions. The husband feels that he is doing everything in his power to pay attention and listen to his wife. His wife's nervous system is sensitive to auditory input and interprets her husband's actions as "annoying" and a sign of inattention.

The **Sensory-Motor Preference Checklist** [fig. 3] offers a way for adults to understand what strategies their own nervous systems employ to achieve and maintain appropriate arousal states. Prior to filling out the checklist, adults are requested to think of a situation when they might have been in a low or high arousal state, such as sitting in a boring lecture or anxiously waiting in a doctor's office. They are asked to fill out the checklist by placing an arrow pointing up for those items that seem to be alerting to their nervous system and an arrow pointing down for those that seem calming. This checklist is not exhaustive but reflects the typical ways that nervous systems may respond when in low or high arousal states.

"DETECTIVE WORK"

All involved in the Alert Program need to be "detectives". They need to watch for subtle cues from students that indicate what types of sensory-motor strategies are being used for self-regulation, attention, and function.

When looking at a student's behavior (his performance and actions), one first needs to decide if the strategy being used (often misjudged as inappropriate behavior) needs to change. What sensory-motor experience is the student seeking? Is it working? Why would one consider changing the behavior? Is the change necessary for the individual's safety, other's safety, or the needs of the adult?

If change is necessary, the adult should determine which sensory-motor input the student is seeking. For example, a girl is seated at the dining room table, trying to complete a homework assignment. She begins making clicking

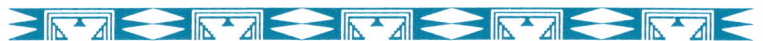

sounds with her tongue. The parent may "detect" that the student is attempting to use oral motor input to maintain arousal for attention. The parent understands that one cannot take away a sensory-motor strategy without replacing it with one that works as well or better. When no replacement is offered, the student may choose a strategy that is even less appropriate. If the behavior needs to change or is not working, the adult may offer sucking on a piece of hard candy or drinking from a straw. The adult may be able to ignore the sounds if the purpose is understood. Going to another room may also be an option.

When an adult's nervous system is in danger of sensory overload ("losing it"), it is important that the adult explain this. For example, "I like seeing you concentrate so hard on your homework. It seems that making that sound with your tongue is actually helping you get your work done. My engine is running on high right now, and I need some quiet time. I'm having trouble reading the newspaper while you're working, so I'll go into the den to read." This type of explanation promotes understanding, acceptance, and cooperation.

The Alert Program provides a framework in which adults can observe and try to determine the purpose behind students' sensory-motor behaviors. Through detective work, adults may assist students in finding appropriate and useful behavior strategies that are tolerable to all concerned.

STAGES OF TEACHING THE ALERT PROGRAM

Leaders implement the program in three stages: identifying engine speeds, experimenting with methods to change engine speeds, and regulating engine speeds. In the first stage, students learn to define and label how their "engine is running." Next they begin to learn how to change their engine levels, using sensory-motor strategies, and they identify their sensory-motor preferences. Finally, in the third stage, students learn to monitor sensory-motor input to regulate their arousal state. They master how to change their engine levels for a variety of settings, so they can do what they want to do (learn, work, play) in the arousal state appropriate for that task.

Each stage consists of a series of steps designed to help students reach their potential for self-regulation. In brief, the three stages and 12 steps are:

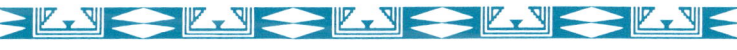

STAGE ONE: Identifying Engine Speeds
1. Students learn the engine words.
2. Adults label their own engine levels.
3. Students develop awareness of the feel of their own engine speeds, using the adults' labels as guides.
4. Students learn to identify and label levels for themselves.
5. Students label levels for themselves, outside therapy sessions.

STAGE TWO: Experimenting with Methods to Change Engine Speeds
6. Leaders introduce sensory-motor methods to change engine levels.
7. Leaders identify sensory-motor preferences and sensory hypersensitivities.
8. Students begin experimentation with choosing strategies.

STAGE THREE: Regulating Engine Speeds
9. Students choose sensory-motor strategies independently.
10. Students use strategies independently, outside therapy sessions.
11. Students learn to change engine levels when options are limited.
12. Students continue receiving support.

A person need not complete the entire program to benefit. Usually, only students who are functioning at a level of eight years or older can attain the self-knowledge to regulate their arousal states without adult supervision. Those who are developmentally younger than eight years of age are not expected to complete the third stage. Rather than incorporate the whole program, parents and teachers may choose to use only the program's vocabulary to identify and label how a child's engine is running, and avoid using words that may have negative connotations such as "hyper" or "out of control."

It is exciting to watch children's pride as they express their knowledge of arousal states. Readers may be delighted to discover the ease with which many students learn the concepts of the Alert Program. The authors hope that the information in this booklet provides readers with new insight into self-regulation, so children can be supported in answering the question, "How does your engine run?"

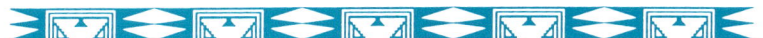

Figure 3

SENSORY-MOTOR PREFERENCE CHECKLIST (FOR ADULTS)

DIRECTIONS: This checklist was developed to help adults recognize what strategies their own nervous systems employ to attain an appropriate state of alertness. Mark the items below that you use to increase (↑) or to decrease (↓) your state of alertness. You might mark both (↑↓) on some items. Others you might not use at all.

SOMETHING IN YOUR MOUTH (ORAL MOTOR INPUT):

__ drink a milkshake
__ suck on hard candy
__ crunch or suck on ice pieces
__ tongue in cheek movements
__ "chew" on pencil / pen
__ chew on coffee swizzle sticks
__ take slow deep breaths
__ suck, lick, bite on your lips or the inside of your cheeks
__ drink carbonated drink
__ eat a cold popsicle
__ eat a pickle

__ chew gum
__ crunch on nuts / pretzels / chips
__ bite on nails / cuticle
__ eat popcorn / cut up vegetables
__ eat chips and a spicy dip
__ smoke cigarettes
__ chew on buttons, sweatshirt strings or collars
__ whistle while you work
__ drink coffee / tea (caffeinated)
__ drink hot cocoa or warm milk
__ other:

MOVE (VESTIBULAR INPUT):

__ rock in a rocking chair
__ shift or "squirm" in a chair
__ push chair back on 2 legs
__ aerobic exercise
__ isometrics / lift weights
__ rock own body slightly
__ scrub kitchen floor
__ roll neck and head slowly

__ sit with crossed legs and bounce one slightly
__ run / jog
__ ride bike
__ tap toe, heel or foot
__ dance
__ yard work
__ stretch / shake body parts
__ other:

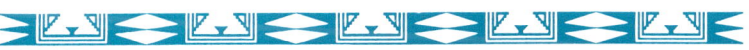

Figure 3 - *Continued*

TOUCH (TACTILE INPUT):

__ twist own hair
__ move keys or coins in pocket with your hand
__ cool shower
__ warm bath
__ receive a massage
__ pet a dog or cat
__ drum fingers or pencil on table
__ rub gently on skin / clothes

* Fidget with the following:
__ a straw
__ paper clips
__ cuticle / nails
__ pencil / pen
__ earring or necklace
__ phone cord while talking
__ put fingers near mouth, eye, or nose
__ other:

LOOK (VISUAL INPUT):

__ open window shades after a boring movie in a classroom
__ watch a fireplace
__ watch fish tank
__ watch sunset / sunrise
__ watch "oil and water" toys

* How do you react to:
__ dim lighting
__ fluorescent lighting
__ sunlight through bedroom window when sleeping
__ rose colored room
__ a "cluttered desk" when needing to concentrate

LISTEN (AUDITORY INPUT):

__ listen to Classical Music
__ listen to Hard Rock
__ listen to others "hum"
__ work in "quiet" room
__ work in "noisy" room
__ sing or talk to self

* How do you react to:
__ scratch on a chalkboard
__ "squeak" of a mechanical pencil
__ fire siren
__ waking to an unusual noise
__ dog barking (almost constantly)

Figure 3 - *Continued*
QUESTIONS TO PONDER

1. Review this Sensory-Motor Preference Checklist. Think about what you do in a small, subtle manner to maintain an appropriate alert level that a child with a less mature nervous system may need to do in a larger more intense way.

2. Notice which types of sensory input are comforting to your nervous system and which types of sensory input bother your nervous system. Are your items clustered in a certain category of sensory input?

3. Consider how often (frequency), how long (duration), how much (intensity), and with what rhythm (fast, slow, uneven or even) you use these inputs to change your state of alertness.

4. When you are needing to concentrate at your work space, what sensory input do you prefer to work most efficiently?
    a) What do you put in or around your mouth?
       (Example: food, drink, gum, etc.)
    b) What do you prefer to touch?
       (Example: clothing, texture of chair, fidgeting with objects, etc.)
    c) What types of movement do you use?
       (Example: rock in chair or movement breaks to stretch or walk, etc.)
    d) What are your visual preferences?
       (Example: natural lighting from window, use of a lamp, brightly colored walls. Are you an "in" person working best with your desk cleared off or an "out" person whose desk is piled high with papers, etc.)
    e) What auditory input do you use?
       (Example: do you listen to music while you work? If so, what type of beat? Do you like to talk to yourself or others and work at the same time? Do you prefer a quiet environment?, etc.)

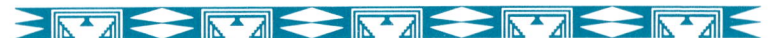

REFERENCES

Ayres, A. J. (1974). *The development of sensory integrative theory and practice: A collection of the works of A. Jean Ayres*. Rockville, MD: American Occupational Therapy Association.

Ayres, A. J. (1979). *Sensory integration and the child*. Los Angeles: Western Psychological Services.

Cool, S., & Oetter, P. (1990). *New treatment perspectives: sensory integration and principles of neural systems organization*. Paper presentation in Boston.

DeGangi, G. A., & Porges, S. W. (1991). Attention/Alertness/Arousal. In Chapter 5 of the *AOTA self study series neuroscience foundations of human performance*. Rockville, MD: American Occupational Therapy Association, Inc.

Fisher, A. G., Murray, E. A., & Bundy, A. C. (1991). *Sensory integration theory and practice*. Philadelphia: F. A. Davis Company.

Kramer, P., & Hinojosa, J. (1993). *Frames of reference for pediatric occupational therapy*. Baltimore: Williams & Wilkins.

Mercer, C. D., & Snell, M. E. (1977). *Learning theory in mental retardation: Implications for teaching*. Columbus, OH: Charles E. Merrill Publishing Company.

Moore, J. C. (1985). *Arousal and attention: Neurological and clinical considerations*. Paper presented in St. Paul, MN: Professional Development Programs.

Oetter, P., Richter, E. W., & Frick, S. M. (1993). *MORE Integrating the mouth with sensory and postural functions*. Hugo, MN: PDP Press, Inc.

Reisman, J. & Scott, N. (1991). *Learning about learning disabilities* [videotape]. Minnesota Occupational Therapy Association. Tucson, AZ: Therapy Skill Builders.

Royeen, C. B. (Ed.). (1991). *AOTA self study series: neuroscience foundations of human performance*. Rockville, MD: American Occupational Therapy Association, Inc.

SII (1991). *Caution: Children at work,* The Ayres Clinic at Sensory Integration International (1602 Cabrillo Avenue, Torrance, CA 90501-2819), poster.

SII (1986). *A parent's guide to understanding sensory integration*. Torrance, CA: Sensory Integration International.

Trott, M. C., Laurel, M. K., & Windeck, S. L. (1993). *SenseAbilities: Understanding sensory integration.* Tucson, AZ: Therapy Skill Builders.

Wilbarger, P., & Wilbarger, J. L. (1991). *Sensory defensiveness in children aged 2-12: An intervention guide for parents and other caretakers*. Denver: Avanti Educational Programs.

Williams, M. S., & Shellenberger, S. (1994). *"How Does Your Engine Run?" A Leader's Guide to the Alert Program for Self-Regulation* . Albuquerque, NM: TherapyWorks, Inc.

Zentall, S. S., & Zentall, T. R. (1983). Optimal stimulation: A model of disordered activity and performance in normal and deviant children. *Psychological Bulletin*, 94(3), 446-471.

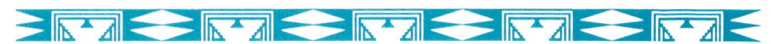

OTHER ALERT PROGRAM PRODUCTS

LEADER'S GUIDE BOOK:
This book is the "original" and explains the Alert Program® in its entirety. It guides you through the 12 steps to teach independent self-regulation with an extensive list of activities and clinical stories. The book includes all worksheets needed for the program.

TEST DRIVE BOOK/CD:
This book, and accompanying CD with its appealing songs, is the fastest way of teaching the Alert Program to children (and adults). The book is full of practical ideas to show you how to use the songs, step-by-step, in classrooms, homes, and therapy clinics.

TAKE FIVE! BOOK:
This book was written for parents and teachers, providing activities that are helpful to keep children alert at home and school. Many therapists highly recommend these low budget, easy to use activities.

ALERT: GO FISH! AND ALERT BINGO:
These printable card games are available from our website so you can print them directly on your home printer. The colorful and playful illustrations teach children the basics of the Alert Program.

KEEPING ON TRACK BOARD GAME:
This board game reinforces the Alert Program concepts. The visually engaging road trip includes instructions and "bonus material" with plenty of tips to make the game successful for children of different ability levels.

ALERT PROGRAM CD:
This double CD set includes an introduction to the program read by the authors. The playful songs are coded for increasing or decreasing alert levels. (Note: these songs do not use the "engine analogy." The *Test Drive* songs teach self-regulation through the engine vocabulary.)

SELF-STUDY CEU TESTS:
Learn more about how you can earn CEU credits for reading our Alert Program products at www.AlertProgram.com

NOTE: Some people believe that they need all the products in oder to use the program. Actually, the Leader's Guide is the only product that is essential for implementing the whole program. But many don't have time to teach the whole program with all its steps and stages, so instead they start with the Test Drive book and CD, Introductory Booklet, Take Five! book, or Alert Program CD. It's up to you! (Go to www.AlertProgram.com to learn more).

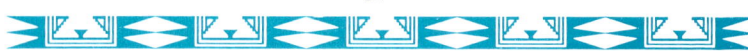